SUPER POMPE POWERS

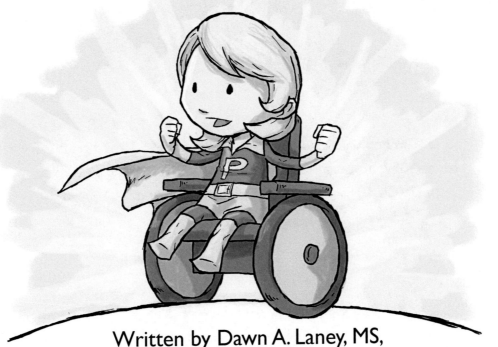

Written by Dawn A. Laney, MS,
Jennifer J. Propst, MS,
and Eleanor G. Botha, MS
Illustrated by Michael J. Johnson

Note: This book has coloring pages in the back as well as a great story to read. If you would like more black and white coloring pages, please contact Dawn Laney at dawn.laney@emory.edu or 404-778-8518.

ISBN: 1479311618
ISBN 13: 9781479311613

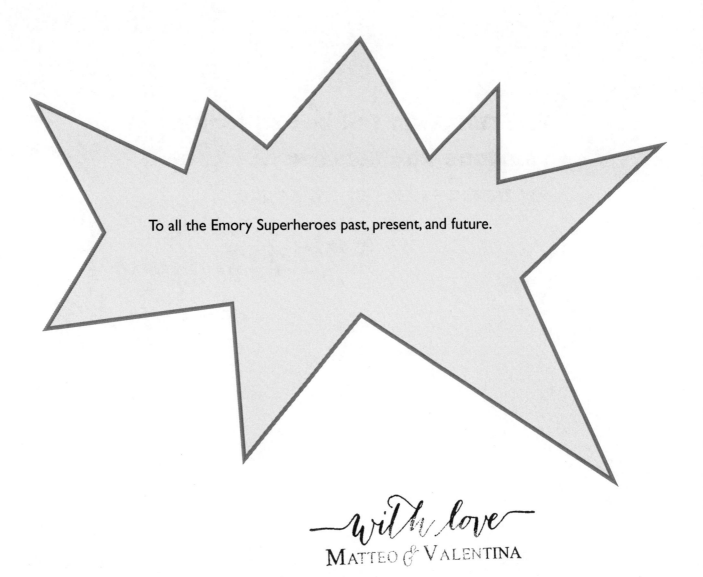

To all the Emory Superheroes past, present, and future.

with love
MATTEO & VALENTINA

You can never tell just by looking at
someone who they are...
My name is Helen and I am a

superhero!

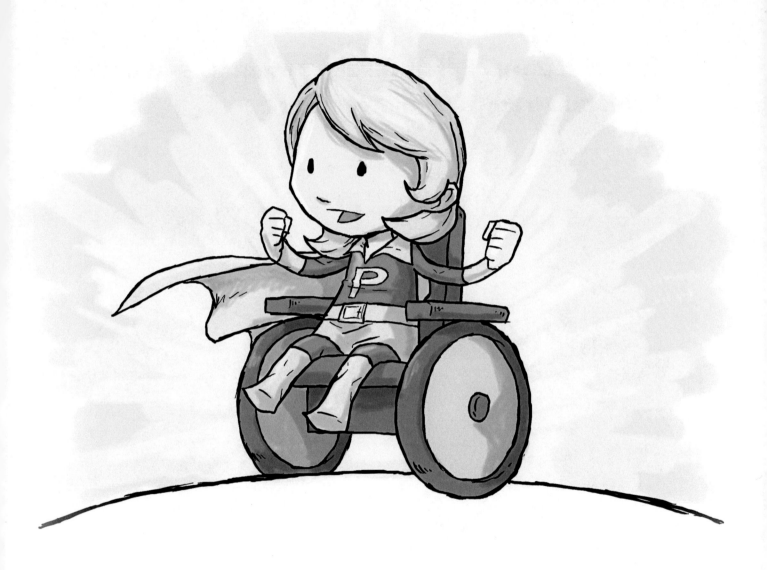

My superpowers are bravery, patience, and hope.
I can do so much with my powers!

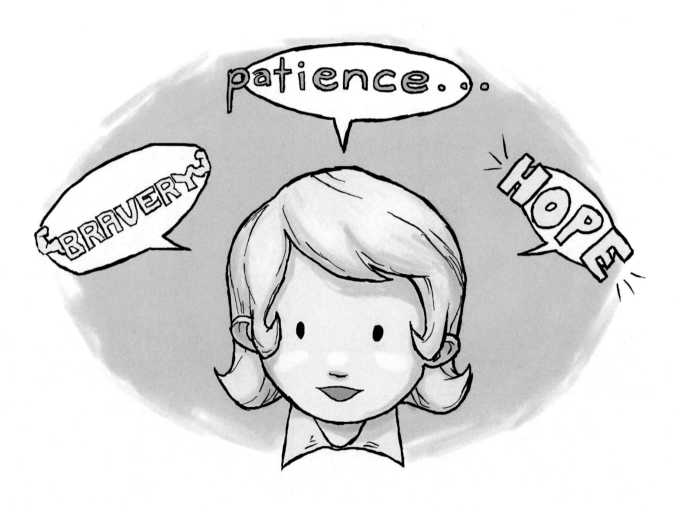

I can lift spirits with a smile.

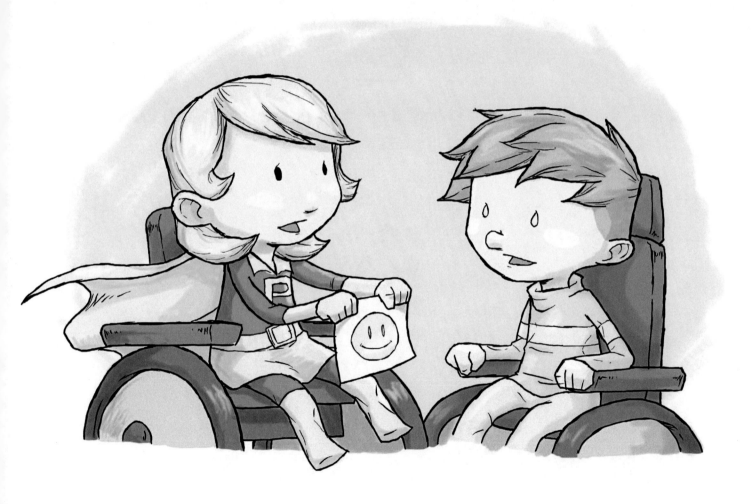

I can swoop in and give those in trouble a helping hand.

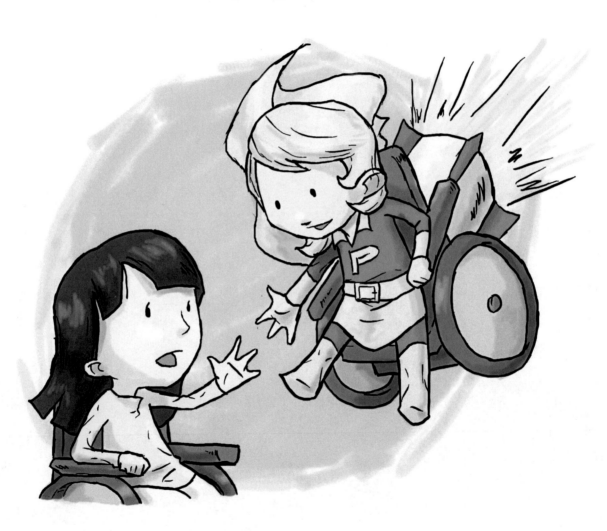

I can help people understand tough ideas.
These are GREAT superpowers!

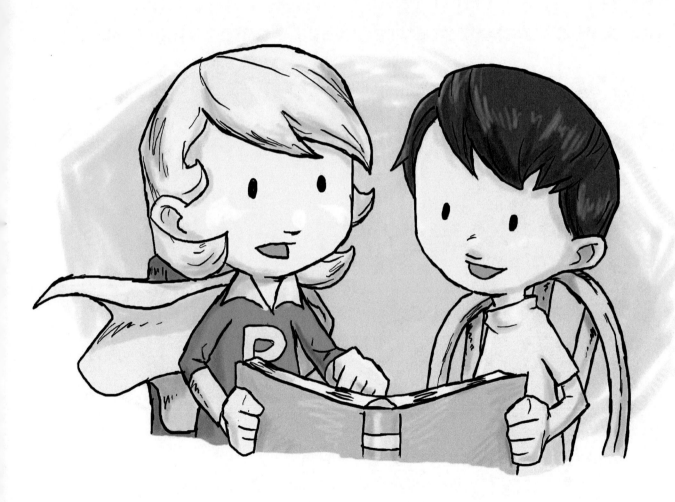

How did I get my superpowers? It wasn't from a radioactive insect bite or being born on another planet.
I am a superhero because I have Pompe disease.

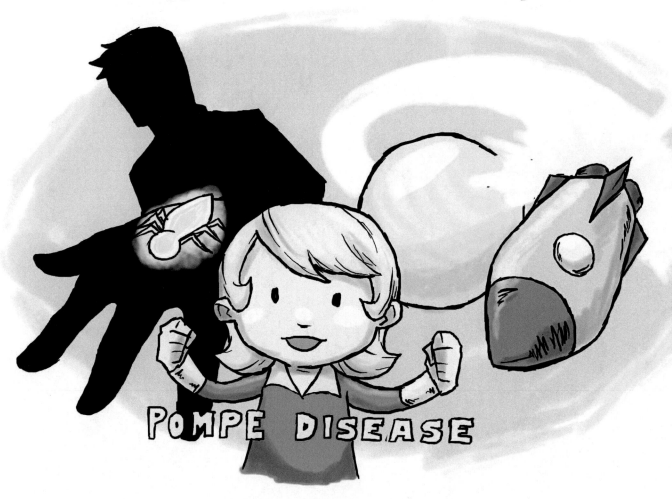

POMPE DISEASE

Having Pompe disease means that when I was a baby, I was very sick.
My heart was TOO big and my muscles TOO weak.
It was hard for me to eat.

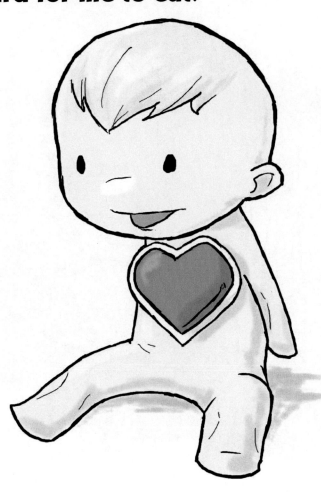

It took the doctors a little bit to figure out what was wrong, but they finally found out that I have Pompe Disease.

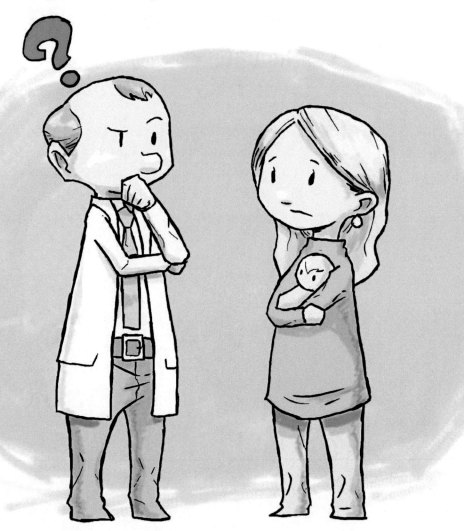

Pompe disease isn't something you catch like a cold.
Pompe disease is genetic condition, which means I
had it even before I was born.
So how did I get it? It's in my genes!
No, not my blue jeans. Genes with a "G".

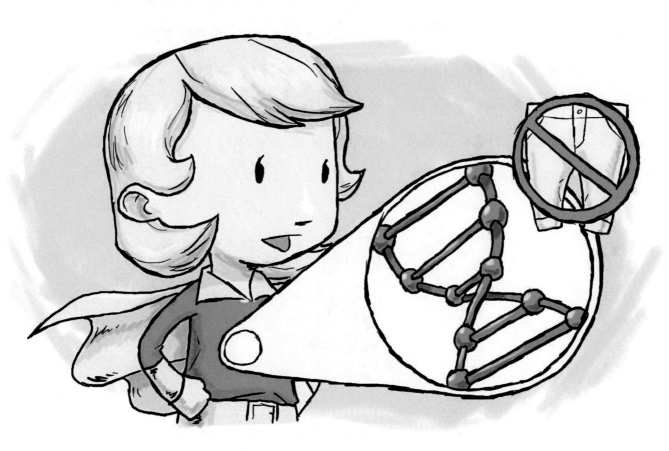

Genes are the instructions that tell your body how to grow and work.

Sometimes you need two working copies of a gene to tell your body what to do. Sometimes you only need one.

The gene named **GAA** needs at least one working copy to tell your body how to work best.

My mom has only one working copy of the **GAA** gene. Since that **GAA** gene is enough to tell her body what to do, she can run for miles.

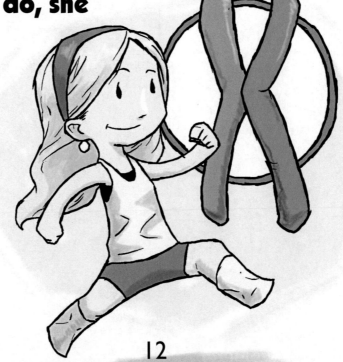

12

My dad has only one working copy of the GAA gene. Since that GAA gene is enough to tell his body what to do, he can push me on the swing for hours.

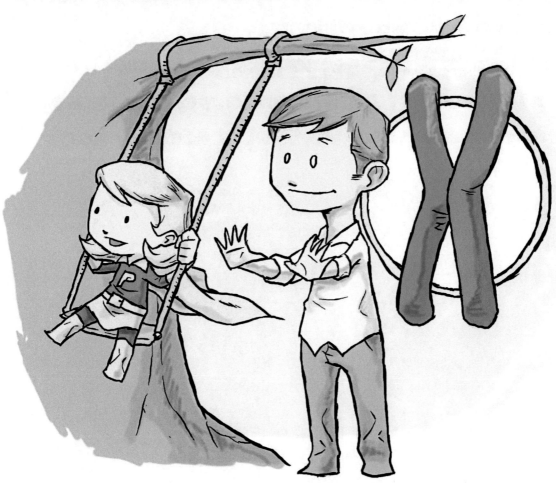

However, when they passed on their GAA genes to me, they BOTH passed on their copies of the GAA gene that don't work. That means my GAA genes can't tell my body how to work and I have Pompe disease.

My parents didn't get to pick which one of their genes they passed on to me, it is just by chance that I have two GAA genes that don't work.

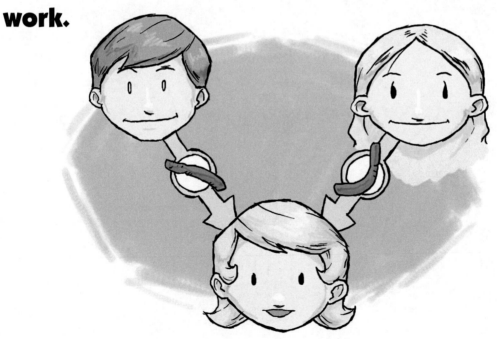

My mom and dad won't always pass on the GAA genes that don't work to their babies.
Look, here's my brother Jacob! No Pompe superpowers for him. He's just like my parents. He has one GAA gene that works and one that doesn't work.

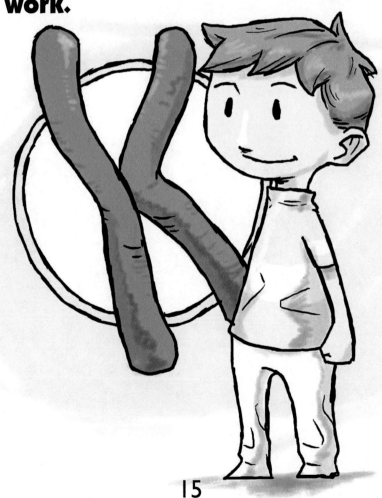

It's like rolling the dice. If I had more brothers and sisters then they could have Pompe disease, be just like my parents and brother, or even have two working copies of the GAA gene.

Isn't that funny?

So what does it mean to have Pompe disease?

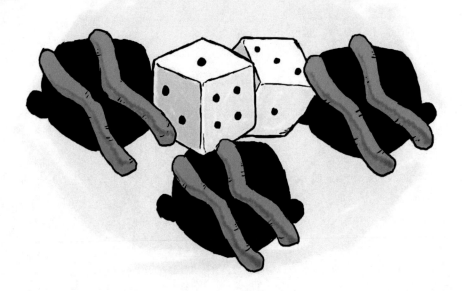

Having Pompe disease means my muscles store a bunch of gunk inside my cells. I can't see the gunk, but it does make my muscles not work as well as I would like.

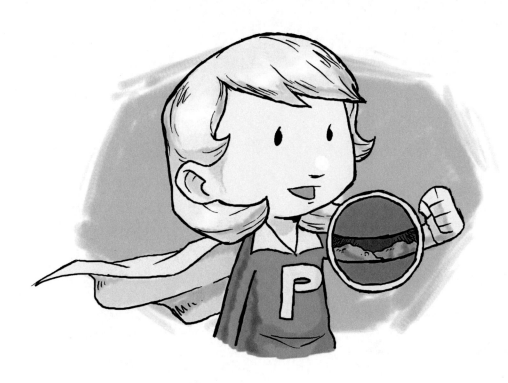

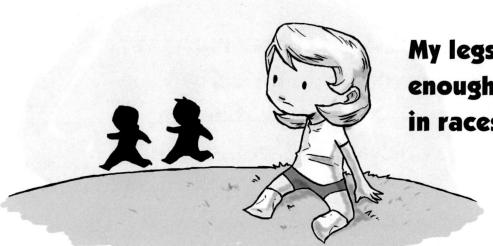

My legs aren't strong enough for me to run in races.

When I catch a cold, it can be hard for me to breathe.

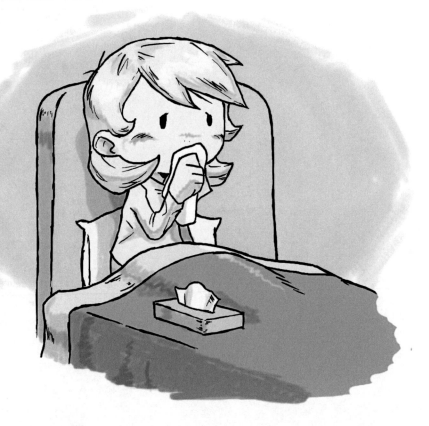

Sometimes my words aren't as clear as I would like.

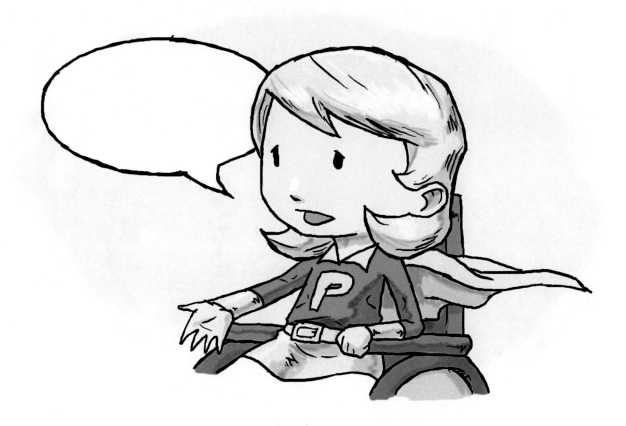

Other times I can't keep up with my friends when they are playing.

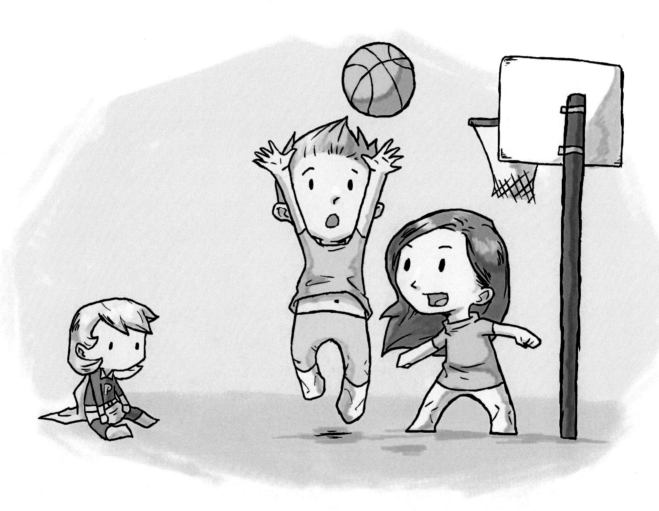

Always, I get sicker easier than my brother.

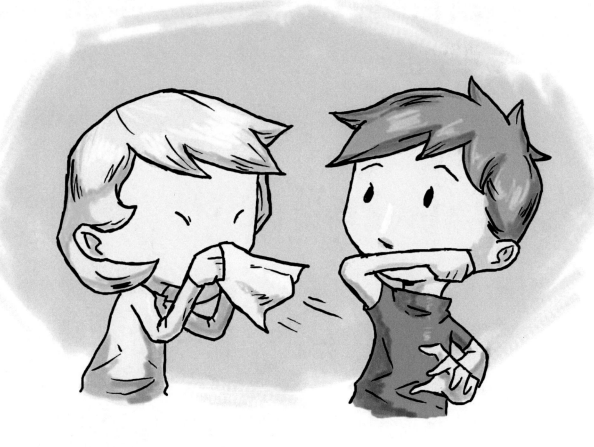

Having Pompe disease is hard sometimes.
BUT having my superpowers helps!
When it is hard for someone to hear my
words, I use my powers to show people what
I mean.

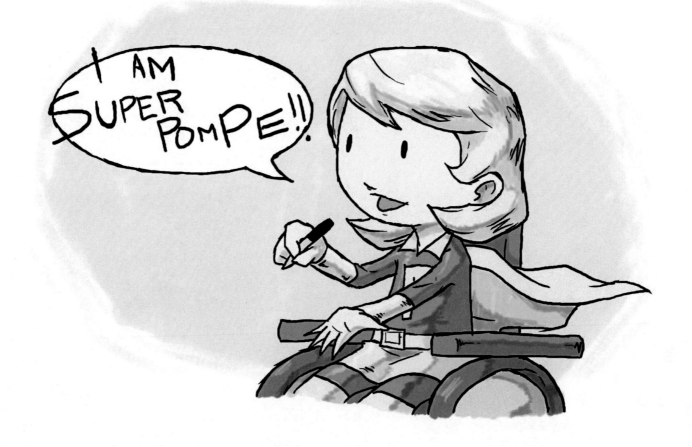

When I can't run, I use my powers to find new ways to keep up.

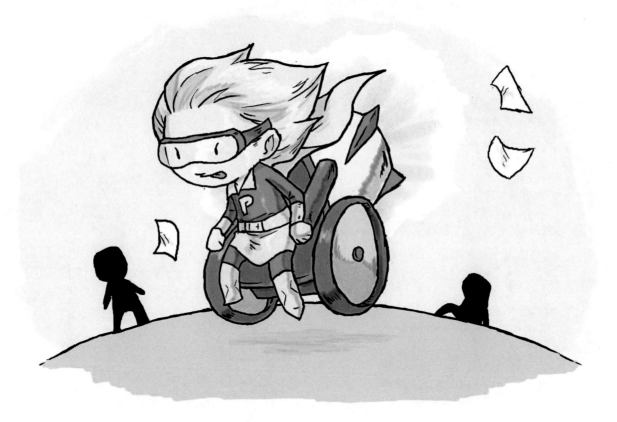

When I am feeling sad, I use my powers to cheer me up.
I use these same powers to help my friends, family, and strangers.

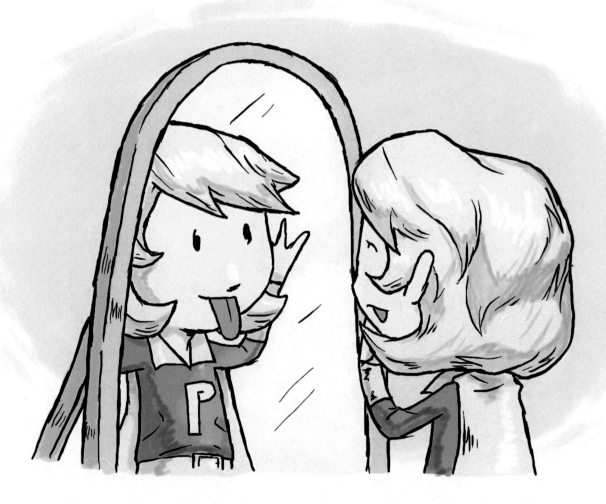

There are other superkids who have Pompe Disease.
They have their own superpowers.

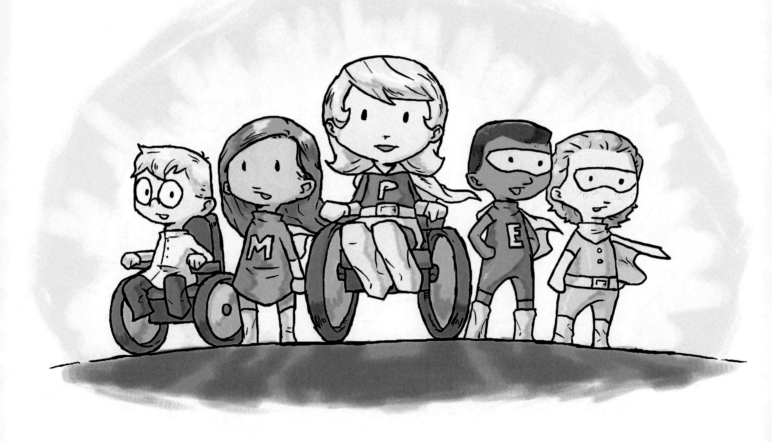

My friend Zach has the power to make people happy.

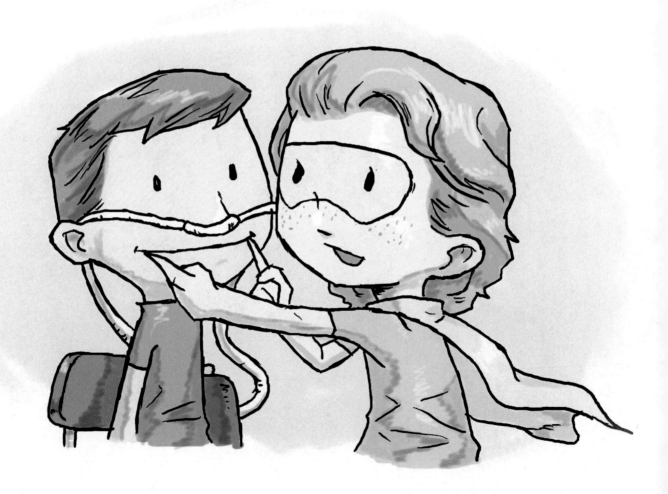

My friend Megan has the power to make things happen!

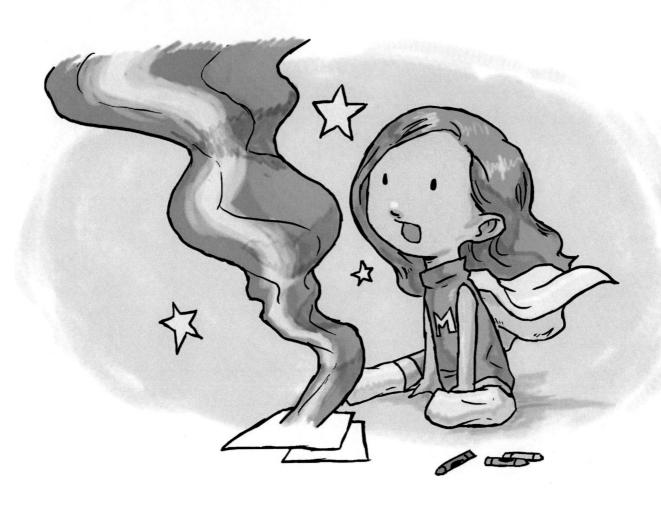

My friend John can figure out solutions
to tough problems.

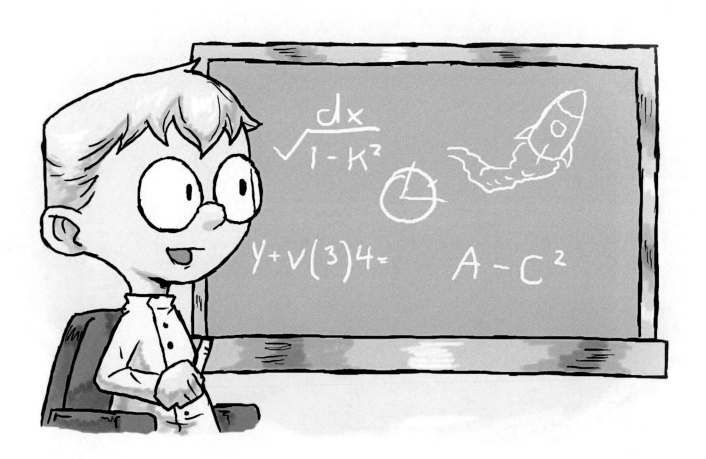

My friend Ethan is brave enough to face a 100 lions!

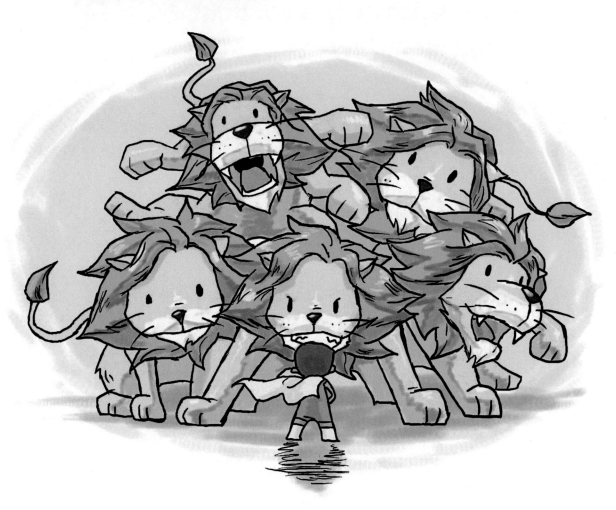

Our superpowers are helped along by something special.
It's not spinach or a bat belt! It's a special medicine.

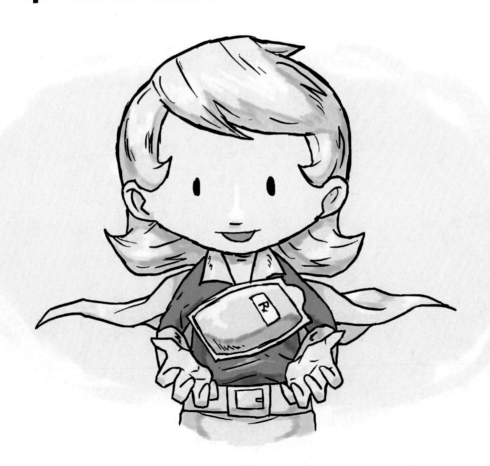

This special medicine is an infusion that I have twice a month. The infusion reminds my body how to get rid of the gunk in my cells.

Before giving me my infusion, the nurse puts a special "no hurt" cream on the place where they will put the medicine.

Then she uses a needle like a tiny little straw to put the medicine into my body. The needle doesn't hurt because of the "no hurt" cream.

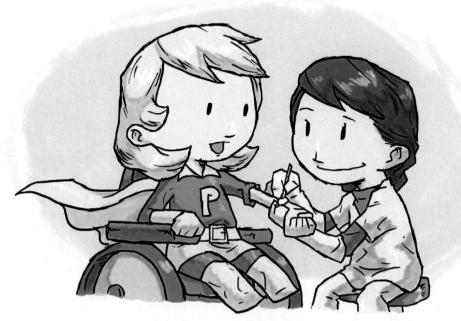

The tiny straw is hooked to a tube and my little bag of medicine.

A small machine moves the medicine from the bag, through the tube and straw, and into me! Sometimes I do need to be brave like my friend Ethan when they start my infusion, but it helps to remind myself that I need the special medicine because my GAA genes can't do the job alone.

Sometimes I get my infusion at the center with my friends.
That's fun because we can all play together.
And they have good movies and video games!

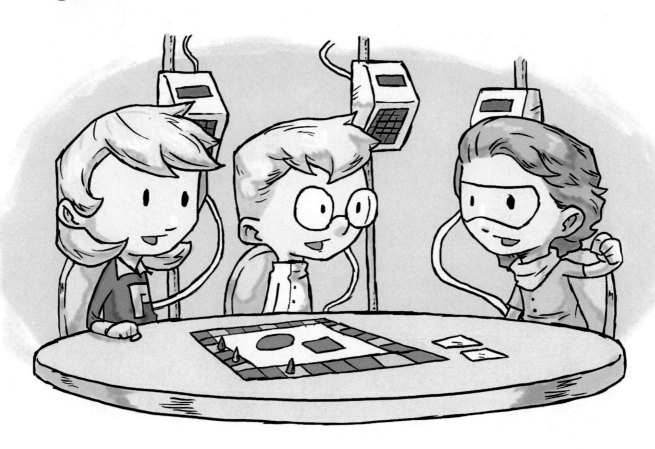

At the infusion center, I see some special people in my life: the doctors, nurses, and genetic counselors that take care of me and help me learn more about Pompe disease.

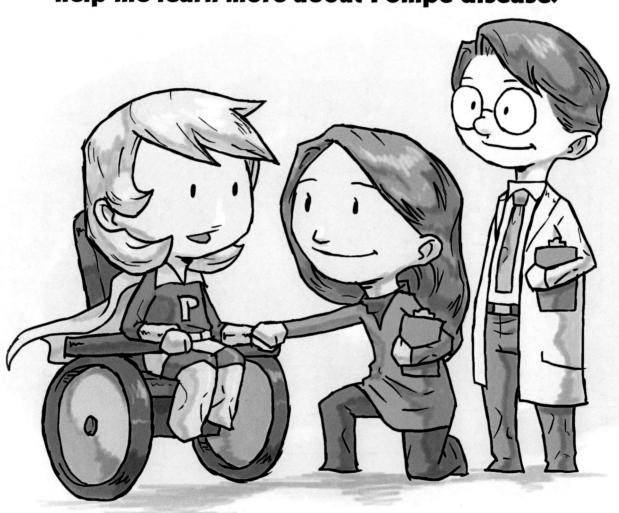

Sometimes I get my infusions at home. Infusions at home are fine too. I can read, color, play games, watch movies, or whatever I want to do.

Even with infusions I still have to see a lot of doctors and do exercises, but my superpowers help me wherever I go.

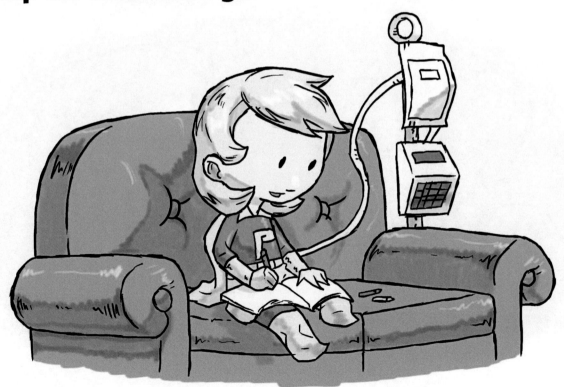

Having superpowers helps me every day, but my favorite thing is helping others learn about new things, like Pompe disease.

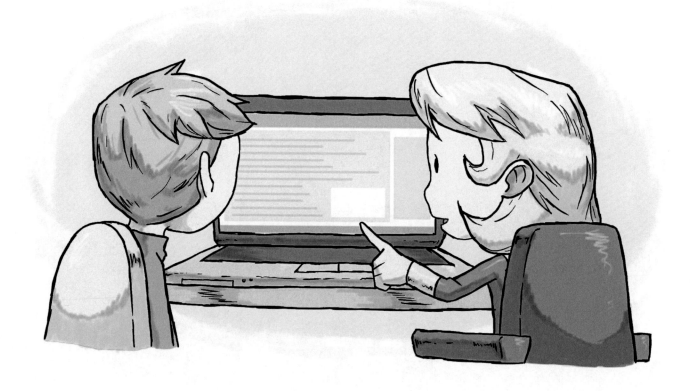

Remember, if you ever need a helping hand, just ask around. You might be surprised who's a superhero. Like me! I am a superhero and I have Pompe disease.

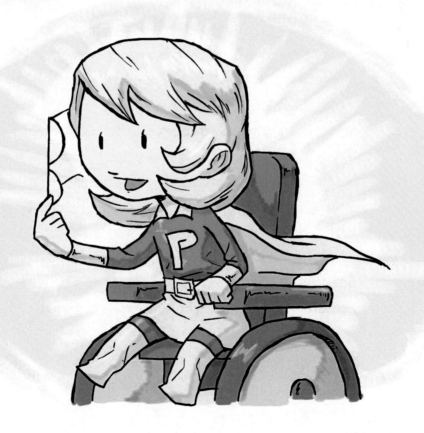

Note:

Helen's superhero story was developed to help explain the symptoms and treatment of Pompe Disease (also called glycogen storage disease type II or acid maltase deficiency) to children. Children affected by Pompe Disease may have different symptoms and therapies than those described in this book.

Pompe Disease is an inherited metabolic disorder caused by the absence or malfunction of a specific chemical or enzyme needed to break down sugar molecules called glycogen. Glycogen is a carbohydrate found in many different cell types such as liver and heart cells. When glycogen is not broken down, it is stored throughout the body within the cell's lysosomes. The muscles of the body are particularly affected. The result is progressive cellular damage that affects physical abilities, strength, and organ and system functioning. Some individuals with Pompe Disease are affected as infants; others are not severely affected until later in childhood or adulthood. The adult onset form of Pompe Disease is often called acid maltase deficiency. All of the forms of Pompe Disease are progressive multisystem disorders with features ranging over a continuum from mild to severe.

Key Pompe Disease Symptoms

The early-onset type of Pompe disease is severe and begins in the first few months of life. The rapid development of Pompe-related health problems occurs from complete or nearly complete deficiency of alpha-glucosidase (GAA). About one-third of all individuals with Pompe disease have the infantile-onset form. Symptoms may include:

- Poor feeding
- Failure to thrive (inability to gain weight and grow at the usual rate)
- Muscle weakness (myopathy)
- Poor muscle tone (hypotonia)
- Poor or absent reflexes
- Breathing problems
- Inability to hold head up
- Difficulties swallowing
- Enlarged tongue (macroglossia)
- Enlarged liver
- Enlarged heart

Some infants and children have a juvenile onset form of Pompe disease with symptoms that begin later in infancy or childhood. In the juvenile forms, early symptoms may include muscle weakness and breathing issues, but not an enlarged heart.

Late-onset Pompe disease (also called acid maltase deficiency or adult-onset Pompe disease) typically begins in adolescence or adulthood. Symptoms of late-onset Pompe disease overlap with those of juvenile onset disease and include:

• Slow, progressive muscle weakness, especially in the legs and trunk, including the muscles that control breathing
• Difficulty walking
• Difficulty climbing stairs
• Difficulty raising arms
• Breathing problems, particularly when lying down
• Fatigue
• Abnormal spine curvature (lumbar lordosis and/or scoliosis)

For more information about the symptoms or treatment of Pompe Disease, please contact the Emory Lysosomal Storage Disease Center at 800-200-1524 or visit our website at http://genetics.emory.edu/LSD

Additional resources can be found at:
Acid Maltase Deficiency Association (AMDA)--
www.amda-pompe.org
Association for Glycogen Storage Disease--http://www.agsdus.org/
United Pompe Foundation-- http://www.unitedpompe.com
Muscular Dystrophy Association (MDA)-- http://www.mdausa.org/
National Organization for Rare Disorders, Inc. (NORD)--
http://www.rarediseases.org/
Pompe Community by Genzyme
http://www.pompe.com/patient/pc_eng_pt_main.asp

Dawn Laney, Jennifer Propst, and Eleanor Botha are genetic counselors and research coordinators at the Emory Lysosomal Storage Disease Center (LSDC). They work closely with superheros and their families affected by lysosomal storage diseases such as Pompe Disease (PD).

Michael Johnson is an illustrator and graphic artist living in the Atlanta, GA area. He has first-hand knowledge of the impact of lysosomal storage diseases (LSDs) on families as he is affected by another LSD, Fabry disease.

Emory's Lysosomal Storage Disease Center in Atlanta, GA provides diagnosis, evaluation, management, and treatment services for patients from all over the United States.

The Center is devoted to remaining on the cutting edge of research and treatment by providing comprehensive and compassionate care for all of our patients affected by lysosomal storage disorders such as Pompe .

To speak with a member of our LSD team,
call 404-778-8565 or 800-200-1524.
You can also visit our website at
http://genetics.emory.edu/LSD

Pages for you to color!

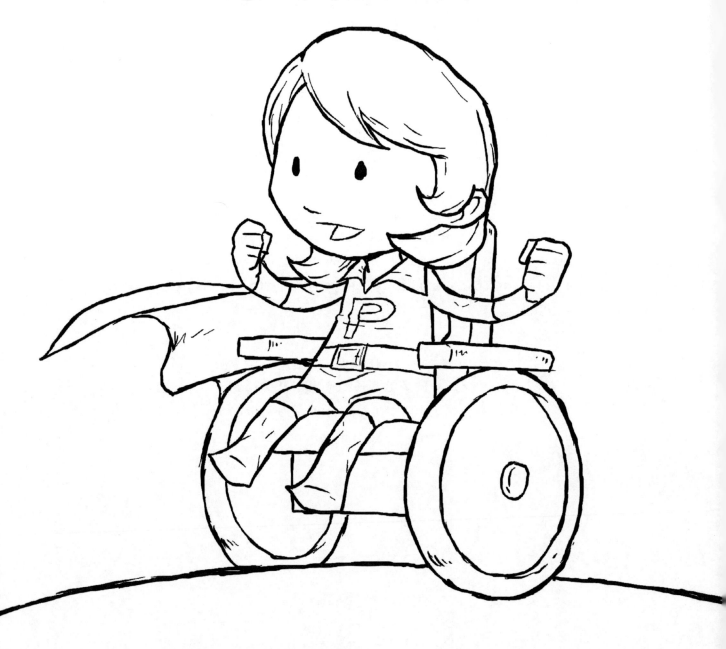

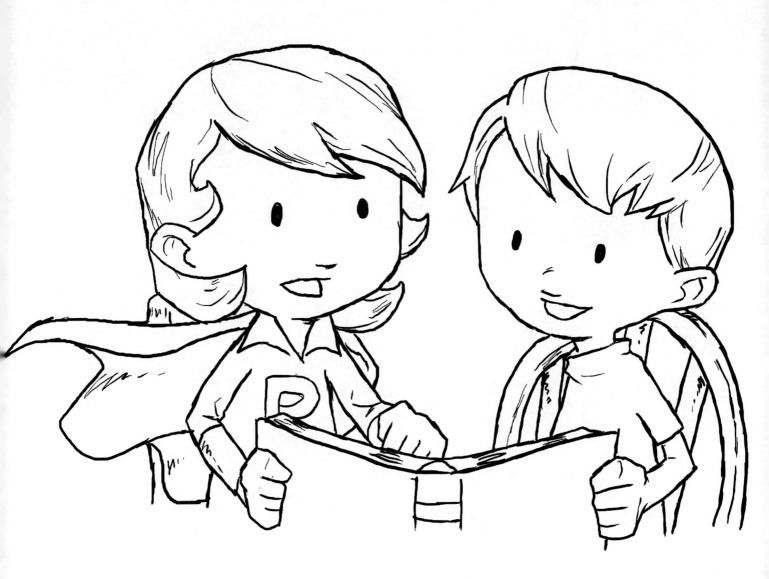

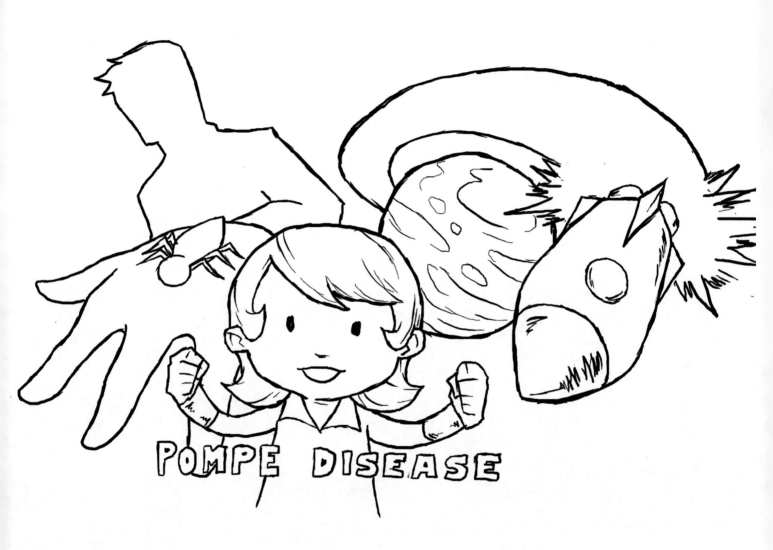

POMPE DISEASE

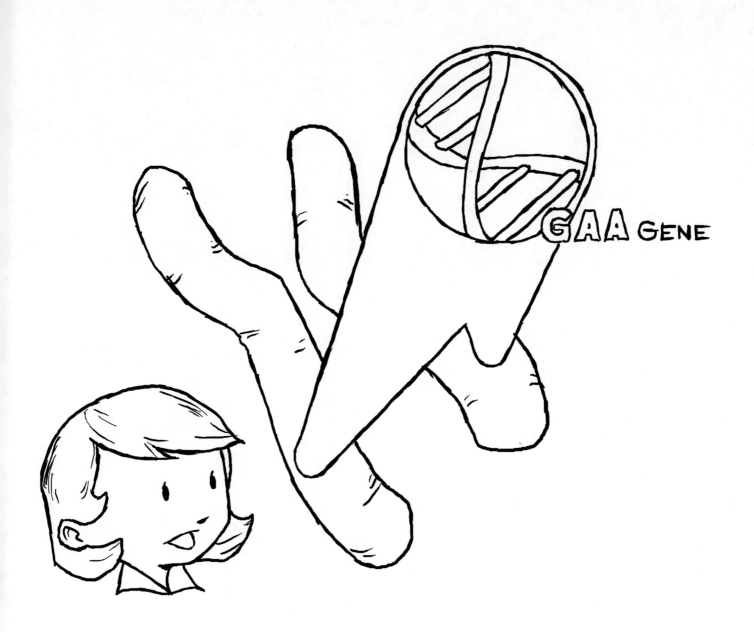

GAA GENE

Made in the USA
San Bernardino, CA
30 December 2015